Thank you for all the long hours an

We appreciate you being the calm in our storm.

Thank you for all the long hours and all your hard work.

_____

_____

_____

_____

_____

_____

_____

_____

_____

_____

_____

_____

_____

_____

_____

_____

_____

_____

_____

_____

_____

_____

_____

We appreciate you being the calm in our storm.

Thank you for all the long hours and all your hard work.

We appreciate you being the calm in our storm.

Thank you for all the long hours and all your hard work.

_____
_____
_____
_____
_____
_____
_____
_____
_____
_____
_____
_____
_____
_____
_____
_____
_____
_____
_____
_____
_____
_____
_____
_____

We appreciate you being the calm in our storm.

Thank you for all the long hours and all your hard work.

We appreciate you being the calm in our storm.

Thank you for all the long hours and all your hard work.

_____
_____
_____
_____
_____
_____
_____
_____
_____
_____
_____
_____
_____
_____
_____
_____
_____
_____
_____
_____
_____
_____
_____
_____
_____

We appreciate you being the calm in our storm.

Thank you for all the long hours and all your hard work.

We appreciate you being the calm in our storm.

Thank you for all the long hours and all your hard work.

_____

_____

_____

_____

_____

_____

_____

_____

_____

_____

_____

_____

_____

_____

_____

_____

_____

_____

_____

_____

_____

_____

_____

We appreciate you being the calm in our storm.

Thank you for all the long hours and all your hard work.

_____

_____

_____

_____

_____

_____

_____

_____

_____

_____

_____

_____

_____

_____

_____

_____

_____

_____

_____

_____

_____

_____

_____

We appreciate you being the calm in our storm.

Thank you for all the long hours and all your hard work.

_____
_____
_____
_____
_____
_____
_____
_____
_____
_____
_____
_____
_____
_____
_____
_____
_____
_____
_____
_____
_____
_____
_____

We appreciate you being the calm in our storm.

Thank you for all the long hours and all your hard work.

We appreciate you being the calm in our storm.

Thank you for all the long hours and all your hard work.

_____

_____

_____

_____

_____

_____

_____

_____

_____

_____

_____

_____

_____

_____

_____

_____

_____

_____

_____

_____

_____

_____

_____

_____

_____

_____

We appreciate you being the calm in our storm.

Thank you for all the long hours and all your hard work.

_____

_____

_____

_____

_____

_____

_____

_____

_____

_____

_____

_____

_____

_____

_____

_____

_____

_____

_____

_____

_____

_____

We appreciate you being the calm in our storm.

Thank you for all the long hours and all your hard work.

We appreciate you being the calm in our storm.

Thank you for all the long hours and all your hard work.

We appreciate you being the calm in our storm.

Thank you for all the long hours and all your hard work.

_____

_____

_____

_____

_____

_____

_____

_____

_____

_____

_____

_____

_____

_____

_____

_____

_____

_____

_____

_____

_____

_____

_____

We appreciate you being the calm in our storm.

Thank you for all the long hours and all your hard work.

We appreciate you being the calm in our storm.

Thank you for all the long hours and all your hard work.

_____

_____

_____

_____

_____

_____

_____

_____

_____

_____

_____

_____

_____

_____

_____

_____

_____

_____

_____

_____

_____

_____

_____

We appreciate you being the calm in our storm.

Thank you for all the long hours and all your hard work.

We appreciate you being the calm in our storm.

Thank you for all the long hours and all your hard work.

We appreciate you being the calm in our storm.

Thank you for all the long hours and all your hard work.

We appreciate you being the calm in our storm.

Thank you for all the long hours and all your hard work.

We appreciate you being the calm in our storm.

Thank you for all the long hours and all your hard work.

We appreciate you being the calm in our storm.

Thank you for all the long hours and all your hard work.

_____

_____

_____

_____

_____

_____

_____

_____

_____

_____

_____

_____

_____

_____

_____

_____

_____

_____

_____

_____

_____

_____

We appreciate you being the calm in our storm.

Thank you for all the long hours and all your hard work.

We appreciate you being the calm in our storm.

Thank you for all the long hours and all your hard work.

We appreciate you being the calm in our storm.

Thank you for all the long hours and all your hard work.

We appreciate you being the calm in our storm.

Thank you for all the long hours and all your hard work.

We appreciate you being the calm in our storm.

Thank you for all the long hours and all your hard work.

We appreciate you being the calm in our storm.

Thank you for all the long hours and all your hard work.

_____

_____

_____

_____

_____

_____

_____

_____

_____

_____

_____

_____

_____

_____

_____

_____

_____

_____

_____

_____

_____

_____

_____

We appreciate you being the calm in our storm.

Thank you for all the long hours and all your hard work.

We appreciate you being the calm in our storm.

Thank you for all the long hours and all your hard work.

We appreciate you being the calm in our storm.

Thank you for all the long hours and all your hard work.

We appreciate you being the calm in our storm.

Thank you for all the long hours and all your hard work.

_____

_____

_____

_____

_____

_____

_____

_____

_____

_____

_____

_____

_____

_____

_____

_____

_____

_____

_____

_____

_____

_____

_____

We appreciate you being the calm in our storm.

Thank you for all the long hours and all your hard work.

We appreciate you being the calm in our storm.

Thank you for all the long hours and all your hard work.

_____
_____
_____
_____
_____
_____
_____
_____
_____
_____
_____
_____
_____
_____
_____
_____
_____
_____
_____
_____
_____
_____
_____
_____

We appreciate you being the calm in our storm.

Thank you for all the long hours and all your hard work.

We appreciate you being the calm in our storm.

Thank you for all the long hours and all your hard work.

We appreciate you being the calm in our storm.

Thank you for all the long hours and all your hard work.

We appreciate you being the calm in our storm.

Thank you for all the long hours and all your hard work.

_____
_____
_____
_____
_____
_____
_____
_____
_____
_____
_____
_____
_____
_____
_____
_____
_____
_____
_____
_____
_____
_____
_____
_____

We appreciate you being the calm in our storm.

Thank you for all the long hours and all your hard work.

We appreciate you being the calm in our storm.

Thank you for all the long hours and all your hard work.

We appreciate you being the calm in our storm.

Thank you for all the long hours and all your hard work.

We appreciate you being the calm in our storm.

Thank you for all the long hours and all your hard work.

We appreciate you being the calm in our storm.

Thank you for all the long hours and all your hard work.

We appreciate you being the calm in our storm.

Thank you for all the long hours and all your hard work.

We appreciate you being the calm in our storm.

Thank you for all the long hours and all your hard work.

We appreciate you being the calm in our storm.

Thank you for all the long hours and all your hard work.

We appreciate you being the calm in our storm.

Thank you for all the long hours and all your hard work.

We appreciate you being the calm in our storm.

Thank you for all the long hours and all your hard work.

We appreciate you being the calm in our storm.

Thank you for all the long hours and all your hard work.

We appreciate you being the calm in our storm.

Thank you for all the long hours and all your hard work.

We appreciate you being the calm in our storm.

Thank you for all the long hours and all your hard work.

_____

_____

_____

_____

_____

_____

_____

_____

_____

_____

_____

_____

_____

_____

_____

_____

_____

_____

_____

_____

_____

_____

_____

_____

_____

We appreciate you being the calm in our storm.

Thank you for all the long hours and all your hard work.

We appreciate you being the calm in our storm.

Thank you for all the long hours and all your hard work.

We appreciate you being the calm in our storm.

Thank you for all the long hours and all your hard work.

We appreciate you being the calm in our storm.

Thank you for all the long hours and all your hard work.

We appreciate you being the calm in our storm.

Thank you for all the long hours and all your hard work.

We appreciate you being the calm in our storm.

Thank you for all the long hours and all your hard work.

We appreciate you being the calm in our storm.

Thank you for all the long hours and all your hard work.

We appreciate you being the calm in our storm.

Thank you for all the long hours and all your hard work.

We appreciate you being the calm in our storm.

Thank you for all the long hours and all your hard work.

We appreciate you being the calm in our storm.

Thank you for all the long hours and all your hard work.

We appreciate you being the calm in our storm.

Thank you for all the long hours and all your hard work.

_____

_____

_____

_____

_____

_____

_____

_____

_____

_____

_____

_____

_____

_____

_____

_____

_____

_____

_____

_____

_____

_____

_____

_____

We appreciate you being the calm in our storm.

Thank you for all the long hours and all your hard work.

We appreciate you being the calm in our storm.

Thank you for all the long hours and all your hard work.

_____
_____
_____
_____
_____
_____
_____
_____
_____
_____
_____
_____
_____
_____
_____
_____
_____
_____
_____
_____
_____
_____
_____
_____
_____

We appreciate you being the calm in our storm.

Thank you for all the long hours and all your hard work.

We appreciate you being the calm in our storm.

Thank you for all the long hours and all your hard work.

_____

_____

_____

_____

_____

_____

_____

_____

_____

_____

_____

_____

_____

_____

_____

_____

_____

_____

_____

_____

_____

We appreciate you being the calm in our storm.

Thank you for all the long hours and all your hard work.

We appreciate you being the calm in our storm.

Thank you for all the long hours and all your hard work.

_____
_____
_____
_____
_____
_____
_____
_____
_____
_____
_____
_____
_____
_____
_____
_____
_____
_____
_____
_____
_____
_____
_____
_____
_____

We appreciate you being the calm in our storm.

Thank you for all the long hours and all your hard work.

We appreciate you being the calm in our storm.

Thank you for all the long hours and all your hard work.

We appreciate you being the calm in our storm.

Thank you for all the long hours and all your hard work.

_____

_____

_____

_____

_____

_____

_____

_____

_____

_____

_____

_____

_____

_____

_____

_____

_____

_____

_____

_____

_____

_____

_____

_____

_____

_____

We appreciate you being the calm in our storm.

Thank you for all the long hours and all your hard work.

We appreciate you being the calm in our storm.

Thank you for all the long hours and all your hard work.

We appreciate you being the calm in our storm.

Thank you for all the long hours and all your hard work.

_____

_____

_____

_____

_____

_____

_____

_____

_____

_____

_____

_____

_____

_____

_____

_____

_____

_____

_____

_____

_____

_____

_____

_____

We appreciate you being the calm in our storm.

Thank you for all the long hours and all your hard work.

We appreciate you being the calm in our storm.

Thank you for all the long hours and all your hard work.

We appreciate you being the calm in our storm.

Thank you for all the long hours and all your hard work.

We appreciate you being the calm in our storm.

Thank you for all the long hours and all your hard work.

We appreciate you being the calm in our storm.

Thank you for all the long hours and all your hard work.

We appreciate you being the calm in our storm.

Thank you for all the long hours and all your hard work.

_____
_____
_____
_____
_____
_____
_____
_____
_____
_____
_____
_____
_____
_____
_____
_____
_____
_____
_____
_____
_____
_____
_____

We appreciate you being the calm in our storm.

Thank you for all the long hours and all your hard work.

We appreciate you being the calm in our storm.

Thank you for all the long hours and all your hard work.

We appreciate you being the calm in our storm.

Thank you for all the long hours and all your hard work.

_____
_____
_____
_____
_____
_____
_____
_____
_____
_____
_____
_____
_____
_____
_____
_____
_____
_____
_____
_____
_____
_____
_____
_____
_____
_____

We appreciate you being the calm in our storm.

Thank you for all the long hours and all your hard work.

We appreciate you being the calm in our storm.

Thank you for all the long hours and all your hard work.

We appreciate you being the calm in our storm.

Thank you for all the long hours and all your hard work.

We appreciate you being the calm in our storm.

Thank you for all the long hours and all your hard work.

We appreciate you being the calm in our storm.

Thank you for all the long hours and all your hard work.

We appreciate you being the calm in our storm.

Thank you for all the long hours and all your hard work.

We appreciate you being the calm in our storm.

Thank you for all the long hours and all your hard work.

_____

_____

_____

_____

_____

_____

_____

_____

_____

_____

_____

_____

_____

_____

_____

_____

_____

_____

_____

_____

_____

_____

_____

We appreciate you being the calm in our storm.

Thank you for all the long hours and all your hard work.

_____

_____

_____

_____

_____

_____

_____

_____

_____

_____

_____

_____

_____

_____

_____

_____

_____

_____

_____

_____

_____

_____

_____

_____

_____

We appreciate you being the calm in our storm.

Thank you for all the long hours and all your hard work.

_____
_____
_____
_____
_____
_____
_____
_____
_____
_____
_____
_____
_____
_____
_____
_____
_____
_____
_____
_____
_____
_____
_____
_____
_____

We appreciate you being the calm in our storm.

Thank you for all the long hours and all your hard work.

We appreciate you being the calm in our storm.

Thank you for all the long hours and all your hard work.

We appreciate you being the calm in our storm.

Thank you for all the long hours and all your hard work.

We appreciate you being the calm in our storm.

Thank you for all the long hours and all your hard work.

_____

_____

_____

_____

_____

_____

_____

_____

_____

_____

_____

_____

_____

_____

_____

_____

_____

_____

_____

_____

_____

_____

_____

We appreciate you being the calm in our storm.

Thank you for all the long hours and all your hard work.

We appreciate you being the calm in our storm.

Thank you for all the long hours and all your hard work.

We appreciate you being the calm in our storm.

Thank you for all the long hours and all your hard work.

We appreciate you being the calm in our storm.

Thank you for all the long hours and all your hard work.

_____

_____

_____

_____

_____

_____

_____

_____

_____

_____

_____

_____

_____

_____

_____

_____

_____

_____

_____

_____

_____

_____

_____

We appreciate you being the calm in our storm.

Thank you for all the long hours and all your hard work.

We appreciate you being the calm in our storm.

Thank you for all the long hours and all your hard work.

We appreciate you being the calm in our storm.

Thank you for all the long hours and all your hard work.

We appreciate you being the calm in our storm.

Thank you for all the long hours and all your hard work.

We appreciate you being the calm in our storm.

Thank you for all the long hours and all your hard work.

_____

_____

_____

_____

_____

_____

_____

_____

_____

_____

_____

_____

_____

_____

_____

_____

_____

_____

_____

_____

_____

_____

_____

We appreciate you being the calm in our storm.

Thank you for all the long hours and all your hard work.

We appreciate you being the calm in our storm.

Thank you for all the long hours and all your hard work.

We appreciate you being the calm in our storm.

Thank you for all the long hours and all your hard work.

We appreciate you being the calm in our storm.

Thank you for all the long hours and all your hard work.

We appreciate you being the calm in our storm.

Thank you for all the long hours and all your hard work.

We appreciate you being the calm in our storm.

Thank you for all the long hours and all your hard work.

We appreciate you being the calm in our storm.

Thank you for all the long hours and all your hard work.

We appreciate you being the calm in our storm.

Thank you for all the long hours and all your hard work.

We appreciate you being the calm in our storm.

Thank you for all the long hours and all your hard work.

We appreciate you being the calm in our storm.

Thank you for all the long hours and all your hard work.

We appreciate you being the calm in our storm.

Thank you for all the long hours and all your hard work.

_____
_____
_____
_____
_____
_____
_____
_____
_____
_____
_____
_____
_____
_____
_____
_____
_____
_____
_____
_____
_____
_____
_____

We appreciate you being the calm in our storm.

Thank you for all the long hours and all your hard work.

_____

_____

_____

_____

_____

_____

_____

_____

_____

_____

_____

_____

_____

_____

_____

_____

_____

_____

_____

_____

_____

_____

_____

_____

_____

_____

We appreciate you being the calm in our storm.

Thank you for all the long hours and all your hard work.

Best Nurse Ever Notebook
You Do The Work of A Thousand Angels – Thank you.
Paperback ISBN: 978-1-989733-18-9
Copyright Dunhill Clare Publishing 2020
All Rights Reserved. Cover Design by Sharon Purtill

We appreciate you being the calm in our storm.

www.ingramcontent.com/pod-product-compliance
Lightning Source LLC
Chambersburg PA
CBHW071431210326
41597CB00020B/3741